REAL FOOD FOR PREGNANCY

"Flavors of Motherhood: Real Food Recipes for a Vibrant Pregnancy"

By

MARY ANN

TABLE OF CONTENTS

INTRODUCTION

CHAPTER 1
- Adopting a nutrient-dense pregnancy diet
- The importance of adequate food for mother and child

CHAPTER 2
- Nutrition of the body: essential nutrients during pregnancy
- The most important nutrients for a healthy pregnancy
- Building blocks for your baby and development

CHAPTER 3
- Culinary fabric: delicious and nutritious foods
- Balanced flavors for the pregnant palate
- Improvement of nutritional value through culinary techniques

CHAPTER 4
- Morning sickness solutions: delicious medicines and soothing elixirs
- Recipes to relieve nausea and increase energy
- Hydration Hacks for the First Trimester

CHAPTER 5

- Sweets for the second trimester: satisfy your cravings at a healthy price
- Making scrumptious, filling meals
- Healthy pleasures for pregnancy cravings

CHAPTER 6

- Fuel for the third trimester: support growth and prepare for work
- Powerful ingredients for the final stretch
- Energizing recipes for home stress

CHAPTER 7

- Postpartum nutrition: supplementation and recovery with the right food
- Replenishment of nutritional levels after birth
- Easy and nutritious postpartum recipes

CHAPTER 8

- Conscious eating for a viable pregnancy
- Practicing conscious eating during the trip
- Create a connection with the body and the baby through food

CHAPTER 9

- Culinary celebration of motherhood
- Create lasting food memories
- Recipes for family and maternity milestones

CHAPTER 10

CHAPTER 11

INTRODUCTION

Congratulations on your pregnancy! You are about to embark on an exciting journey that will change your life in many ways. Welcome to Flavors of Motherhood: Real Food Recipes for a Vibrant Pregnancy, where the journey of motherhood is celebrated through nourishing cuisine. In this culinary expedition, we embark on a delicious odyssey exploring the essence of true pregnancy food. This book is a companion from the first trimester to the last. This book offers healthy recipes carefully crafted to support and enhance a vibrant pregnancy experience. Join me on a gastronomic adventure that not only satisfies the taste buds but also nourishes both mother and child, celebrating the beautiful symphony of flavors that accompany life's wonderful journey.

CHAPTER 1
ADOPTING A NUTRIENT-DENSE PREGNANCY DIET

"Real Food for Pregnancy" is a trusted source that promotes a nutritious pregnancy diet and emphasizes the profound impact of wholesome, authentic foods on maternal and fetal health. Here is a more detailed overview of the principles behind this approach.

1. Whole, raw ingredients

A nutritious pregnancy diet is based on whole, unprocessed ingredients. "Real food for pregnancy" encourages expectant mothers to choose foods in their most natural state and reduce consumption of processed and refined products.

2. Extras containing macronutrients

The book highlights some nutrient-dense foods that are pregnancy powerhouses. From folate-rich leafy vegetables to lean proteins that provide essential amino acids, all recommendations are carefully selected to promote overall well-being for both mother and baby.

3. Balancing Macronutrients

Understanding the importance of balance, the resource guides women to maintain a varied consumption of macronutrients - proteins, fats, and carbohydrates. This balanced approach helps stabilize energy levels, supports proper fetal development, and meets the changing nutritional needs of pregnancy.

4. **Careful combination of nutrients**
"Real food for pregnancy" emphasizes the synergy of nutrients in a meal. By encouraging a conscious connection with food, the book ensures that the body absorbs and utilizes the essential vitamins and minerals that are critical for a healthy pregnancy.

5. **Response to craving and aversion**
Understanding the dynamic nature of pregnancy cravings and aversions, the book offers strategies for managing these fluctuations without compromising nutritional integrity. It offers alternative, nutritious options to suit changing taste preferences.

6. **Individual nutrition**
Knowing that each pregnancy journey is unique, the resource promotes personalized nutrition. It guides women to adapt their diet to

their personal needs and circumstances, taking into account factors such as dietary restrictions, cultural preferences, and special health considerations.

7. Education-based reviews and evidence-based guidelines

"Real food for pregnancy" goes beyond mere dietary recommendations; it serves as a learning tool. Based on evidence-based guidelines, the book gives women the information they need to make informed choices about their diet during this period of change.

8. Real Ingredient Roots

The book contains a collection of recipes made with real, nutritious ingredients. These recipes not only introduce the principles of healthy pregnancy nutrition but also introduce the delicious and rewarding aspects of nourishing yourself during this special time.

Essentially, "Real Food for Pregnancy" is a comprehensive guide that empowers expectant mothers to make informed and deliberate choices about their nutrition. By promoting a deep appreciation of the benefits of nutritious foods, it becomes a valuable companion in the journey to a healthy and vibrant pregnancy.

THE IMPORTANCE OF ADEQUATE FOOD FOR MOTHER AND CHILD

Adequate nutrition during pregnancy is crucial for the well-being of both mother and child. Proper nutrition plays a key role in ensuring a healthy pregnancy and optimal development of the growing fetus.

 For the mother, proper nutrition supports the body's ability to cope with the increased demands of pregnancy. Essential nutrients such as iron, calcium, and folic acid are essential for the development of the baby and the formation of organs and tissues.

Adequate protein intake promotes the development of the placenta and helps the mother maintain the health of her muscles and tissues. In addition, proper and balanced nutrition helps prevent complications such as gestational diabetes and preeclampsia. Real vitamin- and mineral-rich food choices support mom's immune system and overall vitality, promoting a smoother pregnancy journey.

 The effect of the mother's diet on the child is profound and lasting. The first trimester is particularly critical for baby and neural tube development, which emphasizes the need for adequate folate intake. As pregnancy progresses, nutrients such as omega-3 fatty acids found in fish and nuts play a critical role in brain development.

True pregnancy nutrition goes beyond meeting caloric needs; it prioritizes nutrient-dense options that provide essential building blocks for baby growth. A versatile and colorful diet provides a spectrum of vitamins and minerals that promote the child's health in the long term and reduce the risk of developmental problems.

In summary, it can be stated that the importance of proper nutrition during pregnancy cannot be overestimated. The right food choices ensure the nutrients necessary for the mother and her well-being and support the optimal development of the fetus. Preferring a balanced and nutritious diet is an important step towards a healthy pregnancy and a successful future for both mother and child.

CHAPTER 2
NUTRITION OF THE BODY:ESSENTIAL NUTRIENTS DURING PREGNANCY

During pregnancy, a balanced and nutritious diet is crucial for the health of both the mother and the developing baby. Real pregnancy food focuses on providing essential nutrients to support a healthy pregnancy journey.

1. **Folic acid (B9**)
 - Critical for neural tube development in early pregnancy.
 - Found in dark leafy vegetables, legumes, and citrus fruits.

2. **Iron**
 - Important to prevent anemia and ensure adequate oxygen transport for mother and baby.
- Good sources are lean meats, beans, and fortified cereals.

3. **Calcium**
 - Supports the development of the baby's bones and teeth.
 - Found in dairy products, tofu, and leafy greens.

4. **Omega-3 fatty acids**
 - Necessary for fetal brain and vision development.
- Sources are fatty fish (salmon, trout), chia seeds and walnuts.

5. **Protein**
 - Critical for the growth and development of the baby and tissue.
- Found in lean meat, poultry, fish, eggs, and plant sources such as beans and quinoa.

6. **Vitamin D**
 - Important for calcium absorption and bone health.
- Sun exposure, fortified dairy products, and fatty fish are good sources.

7. **Iodine**
 - Necessary for thyroid function and brain development.
- Algae, dairy products, and iodized salt are good food sources.

8. **Vitamin C**
 - Helps absorption of nonheme iron (found in plant foods).
- Citrus fruits, strawberries, and peppers contain a lot of vitamin C.

9. **Zinc**
 - Supports the immune system and contributes to the formation of DNA.
- Found in meat, dairy products, nuts and legumes.

10. **Vitamin A**
 - Crucial for the development of the baby and the eyes, skin, and immune system.
- Sources are sweet potatoes, carrots, and leafy greens.

A true pregnancy diet emphasizes a variety of nutrient-dense whole foods so that both mother and baby get plenty of essential vitamins and minerals. It is important to consult with your healthcare provider so that dietary recommendations are tailored to your individual needs and the circumstances of your pregnancy.

THE MOST IMPORTANT NUTRIENTS FOR A HEALTHY PREGNANCY

A healthy pregnancy requires a balanced diet that contains many essential nutrients to support both the mother and the developing baby. The right food plays a vital role in providing these nutrients. Here are some of the most important nutrients for a healthy pregnancy:

1. **Folic acid (vitamin B9)**
It is important for early fetal development, and helps prevent neural tube defects. Leafy greens, legumes, and fortified grains are great sources.

2. **Iron**
It is important to prevent anemia and support the increase in blood volume during pregnancy. Add lean meats, beans, and dark leafy greens to your diet.

3. **Calcium**
It is essential for babies to develop their bones and teeth. Dairy products, leafy vegetables, and fortified plant-based milk are good sources.

4. Omega-3 fatty acids

It supports fetal brain and eye development. Add fatty fish, chia seeds, and walnuts to your diet for a healthy dose.

5. Protein

It is necessary for the growth of babies and their organs, muscles, and tissues. Use lean meats, poultry, fish, eggs, dairy, and plant-based protein sources.

6. Iodine

Critical for babies brain and nervous system. Good sources are seafood, dairy products, and iodized salt.

7. Vitamin D

It is important for calcium absorption and bone health. Consume fatty fish, and fortified dairy products and spend time outside to get natural sunlight.

8. Vitamin C

It helps iron absorption and supports the immune system. Citrus fruits, berries, and peppers contain a lot of vitamin C.

9. Zinc

Supports normal growth and development. Add lean meats, nuts, seeds, and vegetables to your diet.

10. **Fiber**

It helps relieve constipation, a common problem during pregnancy. Whole grains, fruits, vegetables, and legumes are excellent sources of fiber.

Remember that a varied and colorful diet of real, whole foods is key to making sure you and your baby are getting the nutrients they need for a healthy pregnancy. It is always recommended to consult a doctor or registered dietitian to adapt your diet to your needs during pregnancy.

BUILDING BLOCKS FOR YOUR BABY AND DEVELOPMENT

Pregnancy is a crucial time for the mother and the developing baby. Providing the right nutrients is essential for the growth and development of the baby #039. Consider these building blocks for a healthy pregnancy:

1. Folic acid for neural tube development
- Include foods rich in folate such as leafy vegetables, citrus fruits and legumes to support proper neural tube formation in early pregnancy.

2. Calcium for bone development
- Ensure adequate calcium intake through dairy products, fortified plant-based milks and leafy vegetables to support child and bone development.

3. Iron for Blood Health
- Red meat, beans and dark greens are excellent sources of iron, which is important to prevent anemia and support baby and growing circulation.

4. Omega-3 fatty acids for the brain and vision

- Contains fatty fish, chia seeds and walnuts for omega-3 fatty acids that support baby and brain and eye development.

5. **Protein for tissue growth**
 - Choose lean meats, poultry, eggs and vegetables to ensure adequate protein intake, which is essential for baby and tissue and organ development.

6. **Vitamin D for Bone Health**
 - Sun exposure, fortified foods and supplements can help meet vitamin D needs, support calcium absorption and promote baby and bone health.

7. **Iodine for thyroid function**
 - Increase your intake of iodine-rich foods such as seaweed, dairy and fish to support proper thyroid function, which is important for baby and overall growth.

8. **Dilution of amniotic fluid**
 - Stay well hydrated with water and herbal teas to support the production of amniotic fluid, which is essential to protect and soothe the baby.

9. **Antioxidants to protect cells**

- Eat a variety of colorful fruits and vegetables that are rich in antioxidants to protect cells from damage and support baby and overall development.

10. **Fiber for Digestive Health**
 - Whole grains, fruits and vegetables provide fiber, which aids digestion and prevents constipation during pregnancy.

   Remember that it is important to consult a doctor to meet your nutritional needs. A balanced diet and proper prenatal care are the basis for a healthy pregnancy and the well-being of both mother and child

CHAPTER 3
CULINARY FABRIC: DELICIOUS AND NUTRITIOUS FOODS

Starting your pregnancy journey opens the door to a world of heightened nutritional awareness that emphasizes the need for healthy and nutritious foods. The culinary fabric woven during this time plays a vital role in supporting the well-being and development of both the mother and the growing baby.

1. Color palette of fruits and vegetables

Bring a vibrant spectrum of fruits and vegetables to your plate. Rich in vitamins, minerals, and antioxidants, they promote a varied diet and promote a healthy pregnancy. From folate-rich leafy greens to antioxidant-rich berries, nature's rich palette becomes a canvas for great nutrition.

2. Protein-Rich Foundation

Build a strong foundation with protein-rich sources. Lean meat, poultry, fish, eggs, legumes, and dairy products provide essential amino acids for fetal development. Adequate protein intake supports the growth of tissues and organs and ensures a solid start for the baby.

3. **Whole grain products for sustainable energy**

Choose whole grains to provide sustained energy throughout the day. Brown rice, quinoa, oats, and whole grains provide complex carbohydrates, fiber, and essential nutrients. This foundation helps stabilize blood sugar and promotes digestion.

4. **Omega-3 fatty acids for brain development**

Contains omega-3 fatty acids, especially DHA, which are crucial for baby and brain and vision development. Fatty fish such as salmon, walnuts, chia seeds, and flax seeds are excellent sources that promote cognitive well-being in the growing fetus.

5. **Dairy Products for Calcium**

Ensure calcium intake to promote bone development and overall health. Dairy products such as milk, yogurt, and cheese are valuable sources. If you are lactose intolerant or follow a vegetarian diet, look to fortified options such as almond or soy milk.

6. **Field hygiene**

Stay well hydrated with water, herbal teas, and natural fruit juices. Adequate hydration supports increased blood volume during pregnancy, helps prevent dehydration, and promotes amniotic fluid levels.

7. Conscious eating practices

Create conscious eating habits that relate to your body and your needs. Listen to your hunger cues, choose smaller and more frequent meals, and enjoy the textures and flavors of every bite. This approach promotes optimal digestion and nutrient absorption.

The culinary journey of pregnancy aims to create a versatile and balanced nutritional network. By weaving together these delicious and nutritious ingredients, you not only satisfy your taste buds but also provide your body and your growing baby with the building blocks for a healthy and successful pregnancy.

BALANCED FLAVORS FOR THE PREGNANT PALATE

Creating balanced flavors for the pregnant palate is important not only to provide a delightful culinary experience but also to ensure that the nutritional needs of the mother and growing baby are met. Proper pregnancy food should focus on a harmonious combination of flavors to satisfy appetite and support general well-being.

1. **Sweet and Salty Symmetry**
 - Integrate sweet and savory elements into meals to meet changing taste preferences during pregnancy.
 - Use the natural sweetness of fruits like berries or mango to balance salty foods like roast chicken or roasted vegetables.

2. **Harmony of texture**
 - Different compositions can enhance the eating experience. Add crunchy bits like nuts or seeds, which have a softer texture than cooked grains or steamed vegetables.
- Whole grains like quinoa or bulgur can add a chewy texture to salads, contributing to a versatile meal.

3. **Glow of lemons**
 - Citrus flavors can provide a refreshing and sharp kick. Consider adding lemon or lime zest to dishes to add brightness.
- Citrus fruits also contain a lot of vitamin C, which is crucial for supporting the immune system during pregnancy.

4. **Herbal Elegance**
 - Fresh herbs such as basil, mint or cilantro can enhance the flavor profile of food without adding too many calories.
 - Try herb-infused oils or simple herb garnishes to add sophistication to your dishes.

5. **Umami Enrichment**
 - Add umami-rich ingredients such as mushrooms, tomatoes, or soy-based products to increase the overall depth of flavor.
- Grilled or roasted vegetables can create a delicious umami flavor that satisfies the appetite and provides important nutrients.

6. **Balanced spice palette**
 - Spices can be used judiciously to bring heat and depth to dishes. Choose mild spices to avoid overwhelming your sensitive palate during pregnancy.

- For a subtle and balanced flavor experience, consider cinnamon in breakfast foods or some cumin in savory dishes.

7. **Protein Diversity**
 - Versatile protein sources to ensure versatile nutritional intake. Include lean meats, legumes, dairy, and plant-based proteins in your meals.
- Grilled fish, lentil soups, or yogurt-based sauces can offer different flavors and textures.

8. **Careful use of salt**
 - Use salt judiciously to enhance flavors without excessive sodium intake. Try alternative seasonings such as garlic, onion, or herbs to reduce your dependence on salt. - Choose natural sea salt or Himalayan salt to add minerals.

With a variety of tastes, textures, and nutritional components, real pregnancy food can provide a satisfying and nutritious experience for both the expectant mother and her growing baby.

IMPROVEMENT OF NUTRITIONAL VALUE THROUGH CULINARY TECHNIQUES

Increasing the nutritional value of real food during pregnancy can be achieved through various culinary techniques, where both taste and health come first. Here are some strategies to optimize nutritional value:

1. Steaming and grilling

Preserve essential nutrients by steaming vegetables, preserving their vitamins and minerals. Grilling lean proteins like chicken or fish adds delicious flavor without compromising nutritional value.

2. Coloured Dish

Combine with different colored vegetables for a varied selection of vitamins and minerals. Different colors are often associated with different nutrients, providing a wider range of benefits.

3. Smart Pairing

Combine foods strategically to improve nutrient absorption. For example, combining foods rich in vitamin C and sources of iron improves the absorption of iron in the body, which is important during pregnancy.

4. Healthy Fats

Include sources of healthy fats such as avocados, nuts, and olive oil. They provide essential fatty acids that are important for fetal brain and eye development.

5. Fermentation

Add fermented foods like yogurt, kimchi, or sauerkraut to your diet. Fermentation not only improves taste but also promotes gut health by adding beneficial probiotics.

6. Whole Grains

Choose whole grains like quinoa, brown rice and oats. They provide more fiber, vitamins, and minerals compared to refined grains, which promote sustained energy and digestive health.

7. Herbs and Spices

Use herbs and spices liberally to add flavor without excess salt or sugar. Some, such as ginger and turmeric, have anti-inflammatory properties that can be beneficial for both mother and baby.

8. Correct Cooking Time

Pay attention to the cooking times to avoid overcooking and loss of nutrients. Quick and easy cooking methods help preserve the integrity of vitamins and minerals.

9. **Include Superfoods**

Add nutrient-dense superfoods like spinach, kale, chia seeds, and berries to your meals to add vitamins, antioxidants, and fiber.

10. **Homemade Nut Butter**

Make nut butter at home using a variety of nuts. It provides a rich source of healthy fats, proteins, and essential nutrients without added sugars or preservatives.

By implementing these culinary techniques, pregnant women can not only improve the nutritional value of their meals but also enjoy a varied and delicious diet that supports the well-being of both mother and fetus.

CHAPTER 4
MORNING SICKNESS SOLUTIONS: DELICIOUS MEDICINES AND SOOTHING ELIXIRS

Morning sickness can be difficult during pregnancy, but there are delicious and soothing solutions that involve real food. Consider adding these nutritional options to your routine:

1. **Ginger extracts**
- Drink ginger tea or add fresh ginger to hot water. Ginger has anti-nausea properties and can be a comforting remedy.

2. **Citrus Sweets**
- Citrus fruits, such as oranges or grapefruits, as a snack. The refreshing aroma and natural acidity can help relieve nausea.

3. **Cookies and whole grain products**
- Keep whole crisp crackers or toast by the bed. Eating them before you get out of bed can help settle your stomach.

4. **Peppermint freshness**

- Peppermint soothes the digestive tract. Try mint tea or add fresh mint leaves to water for a soothing drink.

5. Protein-Packed Snacks
- Choose protein-rich snacks such as nuts, seeds, or yogurt. They can provide a steady supply of energy and help curb morning sickness.

6. Removal by twisting
- Add cucumbers or lemon slices to the water for flavor. Hydration is key and these subtle flavors can make it more enjoyable.

7. Smoothie solutions
- Mix a morning anti-nausea smoothie with ingredients like banana, yogurt, and a little honey. It provides nutrients in a delicious form.

8. Life-giving soups
- Choose mild broth soups with lean proteins and vegetables. They are not only nutritious but also easy on the stomach.

9. Small regular meals
- Choose smaller and more frequent meals throughout the day. This can help maintain

stable blood sugar levels and reduce the likelihood of illness.

10. **Lemon Water Ice Cubes**
 - Freeze lemon water in ice cubes and suck them when you feel sick. The cold, subtle taste of lemon can be refreshing.

Remember that everyone's experience with morning sickness is unique, so it's important to find what works best for you. Adding these real food solutions will not only relieve nausea but also ensure you get the nutrients you need during this special time.

RECIPES TO RELIEVE NAUSEA AND INCREASE ENERGY

No doubt! If you experience nausea during pregnancy, it is important to find nutritious recipes that not only ease the discomfort but also boost your energy levels. Here are some real food recipes adapted for this purpose:

1. **Ginger Mint Lemonade**
- *Ingredients*: Fresh ginger, mint leaves, lemon juice, honey, water.

- *Instructions for use*: Soak ginger and mint in hot water, add lemon juice and honey to taste. Chill and serve over ice for a refreshing anti-nausea drink.

2. **Banana Oat Smoothie**
 - *Ingredients*: Ripe banana, oats, yogurt, almond milk, a little honey.

 - *Instructions for use*: Mix all the ingredients into a uniform mass. Oats provide sustained energy and bananas are easy on the stomach.

3. **Vegetable and Quinoa Roast**

- ***Ingredients***: Quinoa, colorful vegetables (pepper, broccoli, carrot), tofu or chicken, soy sauce.

- ***Instructions for use***: Cook Quinoa separately. Fry the vegetables and protein, add cooked quinoa, and season with soy sauce. Easily digestible nutritious food.

4. **Peppermint Tea Infusion**
- ***Ingredients***: peppermint leaves or tea bags.

- ***Instructions for use*** : Squeeze a cup of peppermint tea and drink slowly. Peppermint is known for its calming effect on the digestive system.

5. **Fried Sweet Potatoes with Avocado Salsa**
 - ***Ingredients***: sweet potato, avocado, tomatoes, coriander, lime.

- ***Instructions for use***: Bake a sweet potato, and top with a refreshing salsa made from diced avocado, tomatoes, cilantro, and lime.

6. **Lemon Garlic Chicken Soup**
 - ***Ingredients***: Chicken broth, boiled grilled chicken, garlic, lemon juice, dill.

- ***Instructions for use***: Cook chicken broth with garlic, add minced chicken and finally squeeze lemon juice and fresh dill. Nice and easy on the stomach.

7. **Yogurt parfait with berries and granola**
 - ***Ingredients***: Greek yogurt, berry mix, granola.

- ***Instructions for use***: Layer Greek yogurt with fresh berries and granola for a nutrient-dense parfait that's gentle on the stomach and gives you a constant boost of energy.

Remember to listen to your body and if certain ingredients or smells disgust you, modify these recipes accordingly. Staying hydrated and eating small, frequent meals can also help manage nausea during pregnancy.

HYDRATION HACKS FOR THE FIRST TRIMESTER

Hydration in the first trimester is crucial for the well-being of you and your baby. Here are some hydration methods adapted for early pregnancy:

1. Infuse Your Water

Make hydration more appealing by adding citrus slices, cucumber, or a sprinkling of mint to your water. It adds flavor without sweetening drinks.

2. Coconut Water

Choose coconut water as a hydration option. Not only does it help replenish electrolytes, but it also provides essential minerals, making it a nutritional choice for expectant mothers.

3. Herbal teas

Check out caffeine-free herbal teas to meet your hydration needs. Chamomile and ginger tea not only hydrate but can also relieve nausea, a common symptom in the first trimester.

4. Water-rich foods

Add water-rich foods like watermelon, cucumber, and celery to your diet. They promote general fluid intake and provide additional nutrients.

5. Rehydration Schedule

Set a hydration schedule to ensure consistent intake throughout the day. Consider carrying a reusable water bottle for convenient regular sips.

6. Electrolyte Balance

Balance water intake with electrolytes. This can be achieved by consuming foods rich in potassium, such as bananas, and adding small amounts of sea salt to meals.

7. Rehydration reminders

Use smartphone apps or set reminders to drink regularly. This can be especially helpful on busy days when it's easy to forget to drink enough fluids.

8. Room Warm Water

Some people find room-warm water tastier, especially if you are sensitive to cold or nausea. Keep the bottle at room temperature for easy access.

9. **Hydrating Smoothies**

Make hydrating smoothies with water, yogurt, or coconut water and add fruit like berries or mango for both flavor and nutrition.

10. **Monitor Urine Color**

Monitor urine color as it is a quick indicator of hydration level. A light yellow or pale straw color usually indicates adequate hydration.

Be sure to seek personalized advice from your doctor to ensure these hydration strategies meet your specific health needs during pregnancy.

CHAPTER 5
SWEETS FOR THE SECOND TRIMESTER: SATISFY YOUR CRAVINGS AT A HEALTHY PRICE

Indulging your sweet tooth in the second trimester can be both enjoyable and nutritious. Choosing nutritious sweets can satisfy cravings without harming your health. Consider adding the following options to your pregnancy diet:

1. **Dark Chocolate**
 Rich in antioxidants, dark chocolate can be a guilt-free treat. Aim for varieties with at least 70% cocoa content to maximize health benefits.

2. **Fruit Parfaits**
 Create delicious parfaits with a mixture of Greek yogurt and fresh fruit. The natural sweetness of fruit combined with the probiotics of yogurt makes a healthy dessert.

3. **Homemade Energy Bars**
 Make energy bites from ingredients like oats, nuts, and dried fruit. These snacks are not only sweet but also packed with essential nutrients that provide a constant energy boost.

4. Cinnamon Poached Apples

Baked apples dusted with cinnamon make a comforting and naturally sweet dessert. This simple but delicious option is an excellent source of fiber and vitamins.

5. Chia Seed Pudding

Chia seeds soaked in milk or a dairy-free option make a wonderful pudding. Adjust it with fruits and honey to add sweetness.

6. Frozen Banana Slices

Freeze banana slices for a refreshing and satisfying treat. The natural creaminess of bananas makes them a great alternative to traditional ice cream.

7. Peanut Butter and Banana Sandwich

Spread almond or peanut butter on whole wheat bread and add banana slices. This combination provides a combination of healthy fats, proteins, and natural sugars.

8. Sweet potato brownies

Bake sweet potato brownies, adding nutrients and natural sweetness. Sweet potatoes are a good source of vitamins A and C, so these brownies are a nutritious choice.

9. **Berries with coconut foam**

Add mixed berries to a bowl with coconut cream for a dairy-free and delicious dessert. Berries are rich in antioxidants and add flavor.

10. **Yogurt Cream**

Spread Greek yogurt on a baking sheet, add different fruits and nuts, and freeze. Once it has hardened, cut it into pieces for a nice and nutritious snack.

Be sure to enjoy these treats in moderation and talk to your doctor to make sure they meet your specific nutritional needs during pregnancy. Balancing cravings with healthy choices promotes a healthy and enjoyable second trimester.

MAKING SCRUMPTIOUS, FILLING MEALS

Preparing the right delicious, filling food during pregnancy is important not only for the well-being of the mother but also for the optimal development of the baby. Here are some important tips and delicious foods:

<u>Tips for the right food during pregnancy</u>

1. *Nutrient-Dense*
   Focus on adding a variety of nutrient-dense foods, including lean proteins, whole grains, colorful vegetables, and healthy fats.

2. *Balanced Meals*
   Try to maintain a balance of carbohydrates, proteins, and fats at each meal to ensure constant energy and support the nutritional needs of both mother and baby.

3. **Hydrate**
   Stay well hydrated with water, herbal teas, and fresh fruit juices to support healthy amniotic fluid levels and aid digestion.

4. **Small, Frequent Meals**
   Instead of three large meals, consider smaller, more frequent meals throughout the

day to manage energy levels and reduce discomfort.

5. Limit processed foods

Minimize processed and refined foods and choose whole, unprocessed foods to ensure a diverse range of vitamins and minerals.

<u>Delicious meal ideas</u>

Breakfast
- Quinoa Breakfast Bowl

Cooked quinoa topped with Greek yogurt, fresh berries, and a sprinkle of nuts for a protein-packed start to the day.

Lunch
- Salmon and avocado wrap

Whole grain wrap with grilled salmon, avocado slices, leafy greens, and a drizzle of olive oil.

Snack
- Greek Yogurt Parfait

Greek yogurt is layered with granola and mixed fruit for a satisfying calcium-rich snack.

Dinner
- Vegetable stir-fry with tofu

Colorful stir-fried vegetables and tofu over brown rice, seasoned with ginger, garlic, and low-sodium soy sauce.

Dessert
- ***Chia Seed Pudding***

Mix all kinds of seeds with milk, honey, and vanilla extract, refrigerate overnight, and add to fresh fruit for a delicious and nutritious dessert.

Example of a daily meal plan

1. ***Breakfast***: Quinoa breakfast bowl

2. ***Morning snack***: fresh fruit (eg apple slices with nut butter)

3. ***Lunch***: Salmon avocado wrap with a side of mixed greens

4. ***Afternoon snack***: Greek yogurt parfait

5. ***Dinner***: Cook a vegetable roast with tofu over brown rice

6. ***Dessert***: Chia seed pudding with berries

Be sure to consult a doctor or nutritionist to adjust your meals to your needs during pregnancy. Enjoy these delicious and filling meals while nourishing you and your growing baby with real, healthy food.

HEALTHY PLEASURES FOR PREGNANCY CRAVINGS

Enjoying healthy treats during pregnancy can satisfy cravings while nourishing you and your baby. Choose nutrient-dense options like fresh fruit, yogurt with granola, or a smoothie with leafy greens. Whole grains like quinoa or oats can provide sustained energy. Including lean proteins such as roasted chicken or beans supports fetal development. Treat yourself to dark chocolate because it contains antioxidants. Satisfying your pregnancy cravings with real, nutritious food is a great way to nourish you and your baby. Enjoy these healthy treats to satisfy your cravings while supporting your well-being:

1. **Fruit Happiness**
 - Satisfy your sweet tooth with fresh fruits that contain a lot of vitamins and fibers.
- Choose a colorful fruit salad or smoothie as a refreshing treat.

2. **Nutritious Nuts**
 - Enjoy a handful of nuts for a satisfying crunch and a dose of essential nutrients.
- Almonds, walnuts, and pistachios are great choices.

3. **Yogurt treat**
 - For a creamy and protein-rich snack, choose plain Greek yogurt.
 - Enhance it with fresh berries or a drizzle of honey for natural sweetness.

4. **Avocado Love**
 - Do you want something creamy? Enjoy nutrient-dense avocados.
 - Spread avocado on whole grain toast or add to salads.

5. **The joy of dark chocolate**
 - Satisfy chocolate cravings with dark chocolate with a higher cocoa content.
 - Enjoy in moderation for antioxidants and mood enhancement.

6. **Oat Convention**
 - Warm, hearty oatmeal is a comforting choice that provides sustained energy.
 - Add fruit, nuts, and a little cinnamon to add flavor.

7. **Hydration infusions**
 - Add sliced fruits, such as citrus or berries, to water for a tasty and hydrating alternative.   - It

is important to stay well hydrated during pregnancy.

8. **Cheese please**
 - Satisfy salty cravings with small portions of high-quality cheese.
- Pair it with whole grain crackers for a balanced snack.

9. **Homemade Popcorn**
 - Make your popcorn satisfying and whole grain.
 - Drizzle a little olive oil on top and sprinkle nutritional yeast to add flavor.

10. **Vegetable Sweets**
 - Roasted vegetables or vegetable sticks with hummus can be a satisfying and nutritious option.
 - For variety, try different spices.

Remember that eating the right and healthy foods during pregnancy will not only satisfy your cravings but also provide essential nutrients for your baby's optimal development. Enjoy these healthy treats to make your journey to motherhood even more amazing.

CHAPTER 6
FUEL FOR THE THIRD TRIMESTER:SUPPORT GROWTH AND PREPARE FOR WORK

In the third trimester of pregnancy, providing essential nutrients becomes crucial to support both maternal health and fetal growth. Real food choices play a significant role in ensuring a well-rounded diet. Here are key components for fueling the third trimester:

1. **Protein-Rich Foods**

Protein is vital for the development of the baby's organs and tissues. Include lean meats, poultry, fish, eggs, legumes, and dairy in your diet to meet the increased protein requirements during this stage.

2. **Calcium Sources**

Calcium is essential for the baby's bone development and maintaining the mother's bone health. Incorporate dairy products, leafy greens, and fortified foods to meet the recommended daily intake.

3. **Iron-Boosting Foods**

Iron is crucial for preventing anemia and supporting the increased blood volume during pregnancy. Choose iron-rich foods such as lean meats, beans, lentils, and fortified cereals.

4. Omega-3 fatty acids

Omega-3 promotes the development of the baby's brain and eyes. Add fatty fish (such as salmon), chia seeds, flax seeds, and walnuts to your diet to get a healthy dose of these essential fatty acids.

5. Fiber-containing options

Constipation is common during pregnancy and fiber can help relieve this problem. Whole grains, fruits, vegetables, and legumes are great sources of fiber, which also helps with overall digestion.

6. Stay hydrated

Hydration is essential to maintain amniotic fluid levels and support the increased blood volume. Try to drink at least 8-10 glasses of water a day and include hydrating foods like watermelon and cucumber.

7. Rich vitamin options

Make sure you get plenty of vitamins, including folic acid, vitamin C, and vitamin D. Good sources are green leafy vegetables, citrus fruits, and fortified milk or plant-based milk.

8. **Eat Smart**

Choose nutritious snacks such as yogurt with berries, a handful of nuts, or a piece of whole fruit. These choices provide sustained energy and can help manage hunger between meals.

9. **Balanced Meals**

Aim for well-balanced meals that include a variety of food groups. This approach ensures a diverse range of nutrients, supporting both the mother and the developing baby.

10. **Contact a doctor**

Individual nutritional needs may vary. It is important to consult with your healthcare provider or registered dietitian to tailor dietary recommendations to your specific needs and health status.

By focusing on real, nutrient-dense foods, you can optimize your nutrition for the third trimester and provide the necessary support for the mother's well-being and the baby's growth.

POWERFUL INGREDIENTS FOR THE FINAL STRETCH

Approaching the last stage of pregnancy, it is important to prioritize real and nutritious food that supports both your well-being and the optimal development of your baby. Here are some powerful ingredients for this important step:

1. Salmon

Full of omega-3 fatty acids, salmon promotes the development of the baby's brain and eyes. It is also a good source of quality protein.

2. Leafy greens

Spinach, kale and other leafy greens are rich in important vitamins and minerals such as folate, iron, and calcium. These nutrients are essential for your baby's growth and overall health.

3. Avocado

Avocado is a nutritional powerhouse and contains healthy monounsaturated fats that are important for baby and brain development. They also provide potassium, vitamin K, and folate.

4. **Eggs**

An excellent source of protein, eggs also contain choline, an important nutrient for baby and brain development. Make sure they are fully cooked to avoid foodborne illnesses.

5. **Greek Yogurt**

Full of protein and probiotics, Greek yogurt supports digestion and helps maintain a healthy balance of gut bacteria. It is also a good source of calcium.

6. **Berries**

Blueberries, strawberries, and raspberries contain lots of antioxidants, vitamins, and fiber. They promote a healthy immune system and aid digestion.

7. **Folate protein (chicken, turkey, tofu)**

Protein is essential for the development of a baby's organs, muscles, and tissues #039. Choose low-fat sources to ensure you get the nutrients you need without excess saturated fat.

8. **Quinoa**

A complete source of protein, quinoa contains all the essential amino acids. It is also rich in fiber, iron, and magnesium, which provide sustained energy and support circulation.

9. **Sweet potatoes**

Sweet potatoes containing beta-carotene promote the healthy development of the fetus. They also provide a good source of fiber and vitamin C.

10. **Nuts and Seeds**

Almonds, walnuts, chia seeds, and flax seeds provide a healthy dose of omega-3 fatty acids, fiber, and essential minerals. They are perfect as a snack and a meal supplement.

Remember to stay well hydrated, prioritize whole foods, and ask your healthcare provider for personalized advice based on your specific needs and circumstances.

ENERGIZING RECIPES FOR HOME STRESS

Boost your energy and combat stress with these energizing recipes tailored for home and designed with the goodness of real food, perfect for pregnancy:

1. **Quinoa Power Bowl**
 - Combine cooked quinoa with a medley of colorful vegetables like bell peppers, cherry tomatoes, and spinach.

 - Top it with grilled chicken or tofu for protein.

 - Drizzle with a zesty lemon-tahini dressing for an extra burst of flavor.

2. **Berry Blast Smoothie**
 - Mix berries (strawberries, blueberries, and raspberries) with Greek yogurt and almond milk.

 - Add a tablespoon of chia seeds for more omega-3 fatty acids and fiber.

3. **Salmon Avocado Wrap**
 - Roll grilled salmon, avocado slices, and fresh vegetables into a whole wheat pie.

- Top with sesame seeds and a drizzle of soy sauce for a nutritious and satisfying meal.

4. **Buddha Bowl of Sweet Potatoes and Chickpeas**
 - Roast sweet potato cubes and chickpeas with olive oil and your favorite spices.

- Serve with quinoa or brown rice and garnish with fresh herbs and a drizzle of balsamic glaze.

5. **Mango Tango Salad**
 - Mix chunks of mango, cucumber, and jicama for a refreshing salad.

- Add grilled shrimp or shredded chicken for protein.

- Dress up with lime juice and chili for a tropical boost.

6. **Energy Boosting Trail Mix**
 - Create a mix of nuts, seeds, and dried fruits such as almonds, walnuts, pumpkin seeds, and apricots.

- Keep a can handy for a quick, nutritious snack to keep energy levels constant.

7. **Chicken breast with spinach and feta stuffing**

 - Stuff the chicken breasts with roasted spinach, feta cheese and garlic.

- Fry until the chicken is cooked for a delicious and protein-rich dish.

Remember to ask your healthcare provider for personal nutrition advice during pregnancy. These recipes offer a delicious way to fuel your body and boost your energy levels while relaxing at home.

CHAPTER 7
POSTPARTUM NUTRITION: SUPPLEMENTATION AND RECOVERY WITH THE RIGHT FOOD

Postpartum nutrition plays a crucial role in supporting a woman and recovering from childbirth. Adequate nutrition is essential to replenish nutrient stores, promote healing, and maintain energy levels during this demanding time. Here's a postpartum nutrition guide that focuses on supplements and the right foods for recovery:

1. High protein foods
 - Include lean protein sources such as poultry, fish, beans, and legumes to support tissue repair and muscle recovery.

2. Essential fatty acids
 - Omega-3 fatty acids found in fish, flaxseeds and chia seeds promote brain activity and can help ease postpartum mood swings.

3. Iron-rich foods
 - Iron is essential to replace blood lost during childbirth. Eat more iron-rich foods such as lean meats, spinach, and fortified cereals.

4. Calcium for bone health
 - Dairy products, fortified plant-based milk, and leafy vegetables provide calcium, which is needed for bone health and nursing mothers.

5. Hydration:
 - Staying well hydrated is important, especially if you are breastfeeding. Water, herbal teas, and hydrating foods such as watermelon boost fluid balance.

6. Postpartum nutritional supplements
 - Consider nutritional supplements tailored to postpartum needs, including vitamin D, calcium, and omega-3. Ask a doctor for personal advice.

7. Whole grain
 - Choose whole grains such as quinoa, brown rice, and oats to provide sustained energy and support digestion.

8. Fruits and vegetables
 - A colorful selection of fruits and vegetables guarantees various vitamins and minerals that support general health and the functioning of the immune system.

9. Mindful eating

- Focus on a balanced, nutrient-dense diet. Mindful eating promotes digestion and helps prevent overeating.

10. **Add herbs and spices**
- Include herbs such as ginger and turmeric, known for their anti-inflammatory properties, to aid recovery.

11. **Prioritize self-care**
- Adequate nutrition is complemented by self-care. Make sure you get enough rest and seek support if needed.

12. **Gradual training and movement**
- As your recovery progresses, add gentle exercise and movement to your routine to improve overall well-being.

Remember that every woman's nutritional needs are different, so it is recommended that you consult a health professional or registered dietitian for individualized guidance based on your circumstances. Prioritizing proper postpartum nutrition lays the foundation for optimal recovery and continued well-being.

REPLENISHMENT OF NUTRITIONAL LEVELS AFTER BIRTH

Postnatal feeding is crucial to restore nutrient levels after delivery. Authentic food choices play an important role in supporting and restoring the body and meeting the increased demands of breastfeeding. Rich in nutrients such as leafy greens, lean proteins, and whole grains, it provides essential vitamins and minerals. Equally important is hydration, which promotes milk production and general well-being. Opting for a balanced postpartum diet ensures optimal nutrition, helps restore energy levels, and promotes the mother's overall health.

After delivery, replenishing nutrient levels is crucial for both mother and child recovery and the well-being of the newborn. Authentic food choices are key during this postpartum period. Focus on nutrient-dense options to support recovery and maintain energy levels.

1. **High protein foods**
 Include lean proteins such as poultry, fish, beans, and eggs. Protein is essential for tissue repair and muscle recovery, which helps the body recover from childbirth.

2. **Rich Options for Iron**

Choose iron-rich foods such as spinach, lean meats and vegetables. Adequate iron intake is crucial, especially after childbirth, as it helps restore iron stores depleted during pregnancy.

3. **Healthy Fats**

Include sources of healthy fats such as avocados, nuts, and olive oil. These fats support hormone regulation and are important for a baby's brain and nervous system.

4. **Sources of calcium**

Choose calcium-rich foods such as dairy products, leafy greens, and fortified plant-based foods. Calcium is essential for bone health and can help with postpartum recovery.

5. **Foods rich in fiber**

Choose whole grains, fruits, and vegetables to ensure adequate fiber intake. Fiber aids digestion and helps prevent constipation, a common problem after childbirth.

6. **Liquidation**

Drink plenty of water to stay hydrated, especially if you're breastfeeding. Proper hydration is crucial for milk production and overall recovery.

7. **Vitamins and minerals**
 Eat a variety of colorful fruits and vegetables to ensure a wide range of vitamins and minerals. These nutrients play a vital role in immune function and overall well-being.

8. **Herbs and spices**
 Add herbs and spices like turmeric and ginger, known for their anti-inflammatory properties. They can help reduce postpartum inflammation and discomfort.

9. **Small regular meals**
 Choose smaller, more frequent meals to stabilize blood sugar and provide sustained energy throughout the day.

10. **Limited amount of processed foods**
 Minimize processed and sugary foods as they provide little nutritional value and can cause energy crashes. Be sure to ask your healthcare professional or nutritionist for personal advice based on your individual needs and postpartum considerations. Choosing nutritious, real foods can go a long way toward a healthy postpartum recovery.

EASY AND NUTRITIOUS POSTPARTUM RECIPES

Certainly! Here are some easy and nutritious postpartum recipes that focus on real pregnancy food:

1. **Quinoa Salad with Roasted Vegetables**
 - Boil the quinoa and let it cool.

 - Roast a mixture of colorful vegetables such as peppers, cherry tomatoes, and pumpkins.

- Mix Quinoa with roasted vegetables, and add olive oil, lemon juice, and fresh herbs for a nutritious salad.

2. **Salmon and sweet potato steaks**
 - Mix the can of salmon with the sweet potato puree.

- Form patties and fry until golden brown.

- Salmon contains a lot of omega-3 fatty acids, which are essential for postpartum recovery.

3. **Greek yogurt parfait with berries**
 - Layer Greek yogurt with fresh berries and nuts or seeds.

- Greek yogurt contains proteins and probiotics, while berries contain antioxidants and vitamins.

4. lentil soup with spinach
 - Cook lentils with onion, carrot, and celery.

- Add fresh spinach at the end to increase iron and fiber.

- Warm and rich soup is comforting and nourishing.

5. Avocado and chickpea wrap
 - Mash the avocado and spread on a whole acne wrap.

- Add chickpeas, leafy greens, and a drizzle of olive oil.

- Avocado provides healthy fats and chickpeas provide protein and fiber.

6. Oatmeal with nut butter and banana
 - Boil oats with water or milk.

- Top with a spoonful of nut butter and a sliced banana.

- Oats are a great source of energy and nut butter adds healthy fats.

7. **Egg and vegetable roast**
 - Fry vegetables such as broccoli, peppers, and mushrooms.

- Add the beaten eggs and mix.

- Eggs contain a lot of protein and essential nutrients for postpartum recovery.

8. **Whole wheat pasta with pesto and cherry tomatoes**
 - Cook whole wheat pasta and mix it with homemade or store-bought pesto.

- For added freshness, add halved cherry tomatoes.

- Whole grains provide continuous energy and tomatoes add vitamins.
   Remember to stay hydrated and listen to your body and its signs of hunger and fullness. These recipes provide a balance of essential nutrients to support postpartum recovery.

CHAPTER 8
CONSCIOUS EATING FOR A VIABLE PREGNANCY

Conscious eating plays a crucial role in promoting a viable and healthy pregnancy. True pregnancy food emphasizes nutrient-dense options that support both mother and baby's well-being and optimal development of the growing baby.

1. **Supernutrients**

Focus on whole, nutrient-dense foods like fruits, vegetables, lean proteins, whole grains, and healthy fats. These foods provide essential vitamins and minerals that are essential for fetal development.

2. **Balanced diet**

Ensure a balanced intake of macronutrients - carbohydrates, proteins, and fats. It helps maintain energy levels, supports tissue growth, and promotes baby and organ development.

3. **Folate intake**

Adequate folate intake is important to prevent neural tube defects in the developing fetus. Add folate-rich foods to your diet, such as leafy greens, beans, and fortified grains.

4. Iron-rich foods

Iron is important for increasing blood volume during pregnancy and baby development. Use sources such as lean meats, beans, and dark leafy vegetables to meet these needs.

5. Sources of calcium

Ensure adequate calcium intake for the development of baby's bones and teeth #039. Dairy products, fortified plant-based milks, and leafy green vegetables are excellent sources.

6. Hydrate

Stay well hydrated to support amniotic fluid, nutrient transport, and general body functions. Water, herbal teas, and fresh fruit juices promote adequate hydration.

7. Satisfied eating

Pay attention to your hunger and fullness cues. Mindful eating promotes a relationship with your body and signals, prevents overeating, and supports a healthy weight during pregnancy.

8. Limit Processed Foods

Minimize your consumption of processed foods high in sugar, unhealthy fats, and additives. Choose healthy, unprocessed options to provide optimal nutrition for you and your baby.

9. **Small, Frequent Meals**

Eating small, frequent meals can help fight pregnancy-related ailments like nausea and heartburn and keep you and your baby supplied with nutrients.

10. **Listen to your body**

Every pregnancy is unique. Listen to your body and its signals and talk to health professionals to address any special dietary needs or concerns.

By consciously choosing nutritious, authentic foods and adopting conscious eating habits, you can promote a sustainable and healthy pregnancy and give your baby the best possible start in life.

PRACTICING CONSCIOUS EATING DURING THE TRIP

Practicing mindful eating while traveling is important to maintaining a healthy and nourished body, especially during pregnancy. Plan by packing nutritious snacks like fresh fruit, nuts, and whole grain crackers to avoid hunger pangs and provide essential vitamins and minerals.

Stay hydrated with a reusable water bottle and drink water the entire way. Adequate hydration is essential for the well-being of both you and your baby. Choose water instead of sugary drinks to avoid unnecessary calories. Choose balanced meals when you stop eating. Look for options with a mix of lean proteins, whole grains, and colorful vegetables. Avoid overly processed foods and choose freshly prepared foods whenever possible.

Listen to your body and its signs of hunger and satiety. Avoid overeating by enjoying every bite, chewing slowly, and paying attention to your body's signals. This mindful approach to eating can help prevent discomfort and digestive issues while traveling.

Consider taking prenatal vitamins to ensure your nutritional needs are met, especially if you have trouble finding adequate food options on the go.

Whenever possible, include local seasonal produce in your meals. Not only does it add versatility to your diet, but it also supports sustainable and eco-friendly food choices.

Finally, be flexible and forgiving with yourself. Traveling can bring unexpected challenges, but keeping a positive attitude and choosing nutritious options will make the trip healthier and more enjoyable for you and your growing baby.

CREATE A CONNECTION WITH THE BODY AND THE BABY THROUGH FOOD

The body and the child are closely connected, and food plays an important role in this relationship. When a woman is pregnant, the food she eats is the only source of nutrition for the baby. Nutrients from food are used to build a child's bones, muscles, organs, and brain. It is important to choose nutrient-dense foods that are good for mother and baby.

Creating an interesting connection between body and baby through food is a profound part of the pregnancy journey. Here are the main ways to fix this connection.

1. Mindful Eating Practices

Approach each meal consciously and pay attention to the flavors, textures, and nutrition the food provides. This mindful eating fosters a deeper connection with nutrition and the body and growing life.

2. Listening to your body

Tune into your body's signals and desires. Appetite can sometimes be your body's message about certain nutritional needs. By listening and responding, you create a symbiotic relationship with your body that meets its demands at this crucial time.

3. Create rituals around meals

Creating rituals around meals can make eating more intentional and enjoyable. Whether it's creating a peaceful atmosphere, sharing meals with loved ones, or adding personal touches, these rituals encourage a positive relationship to the eating process.

4. Incorporate Comfort Foods

Incorporate comfort foods that evoke positive feelings and memories. This not only adds joy to your meal but also creates a positive emotional environment for you and your baby.

5. Nutritional education

Understand the nutritional needs of both you and your baby at each stage of pregnancy. The information provides an opportunity to make informed food choices that directly affect the baby's well-being and development.

6. Celebrating Dietary Variety

Enjoy a wide variety of foods to ensure a rich variety of nutrients. Different food groups provide unique benefits, and a diverse diet supports well-rounded nutrition, promoting a strong connection with the body and the life that grows within.

7. Hydration as a form of connection

Drinking water isn't just about staying hydrated; it is a form of connection. Water supports the amniotic fluid that surrounds and protects the baby. Keep a water bottle handy to remind yourself of this important connection throughout the day.

8. Cooking and Cooking with Intention

Engage in the cooking process with care and intention. This practical approach to food encourages a direct connection with the ingredients, cooking and the nutrition provided, which has a positive effect on the body and the child.

By adding intention, awareness, and a variety of nutrient-dense foods to your pregnancy diet, you can create a strong and nurturing connection between your body and the precious life growing within it. This not only promotes physical health but also contributes to a positive and emotionally rich pregnancy experience.

CHAPTER 9
CULINARY CELEBRATION OF MOTHERHOOD

Embrace the journey of motherhood with a culinary feast that's more than just food. Improve the nutritional experience during pregnancy by focusing on real, healthy foods that not only support the well-being of the expectant mother but also promote the optimal development of the growing baby.

Highlight nutritious ingredients rich in essential vitamins and minerals in this culinary journey. Add colorful vegetables, leafy greens, and seasonal fruits to provide nutrients needed for fetal development. From vibrant salads to hearty stews, each dish creates a palette of flavors and health benefits.

Explore the versatile world of grains by choosing whole grains like quinoa, brown rice, and oats that provide sustainable energy and essential nutrients. Integrate lean proteins such as poultry, fish, and legumes to ensure adequate amino acid intake for baby and cell growth.

Celebrate the beauty of simplicity by savoring the natural flavors of the ingredients. Use herbs and spices not only for their culinary appeal but also for their potential health benefits. For example, ginger can help relieve nausea, while turmeric brings anti-inflammatory properties to the table. Practice mindful eating and value each bite as a contribution to the health and vitality of both mother and child. Try meal plans that balance macronutrients and provide a harmonious mix of carbohydrates, proteins, and healthy fats.

Don't forget the importance of hydration. Add hydrating drinks to your daily routine, such as herbal teas and water infused with citrus or cucumber. Staying well-hydrated supports the body's natural processes and promotes an overall sense of well-being. Consider creating a ritual around mealtime, a moment to connect with your baby, reflect on the incredible journey of motherhood, and enjoy the culinary joys that contribute to the shared experience of growth and nourishment.

In this culinary celebration of motherhood, each dish becomes an expression of love and care, fostering a bond between mother, and

baby and the vibrant flavors that promote a
healthy pregnancy.

CREATE LASTING FOOD MEMORIES

Creating lasting food memories during pregnancy involves not only nourishing your body but also savoring the sensory experiences that come with each meal. Real food for pregnancy goes beyond mere sustenance; it becomes a part of your journey and contributes to the well-being of both you and your growing baby.

1. **Diverse Nutrient Palette**

Embrace a rainbow of fruits and vegetables to ensure a diverse range of nutrients. Experiment with different colors, textures, and flavors to make each meal visually appealing and nutritionally rich.

2. **Culinary Adventures**

Make cooking an adventure. Discover new recipes that contain essential pregnancy nutrients. Not only will it excite your palate, but it will introduce your baby to a variety of tastes right from the start.

3. **Mindful eating**

Practice mindful eating practices. Take the time to appreciate the aroma, taste, and texture of each bite. Not only does this enhance your dining experience, but it also fosters a bond between you and the nutritious food you eat.

4. **Family involvement**

Get your partner or family member involved in cooking. This shared experience not only eases the burden but also creates opportunities to bond in anticipation of the new addition to your family.

5. **Seasonal and local delicacies**

Choose seasonal and locally sourced ingredients. This not only supports your community but also ensures that you are eating fresh, nutritious food that is in sync with the changing seasons.

6. **Document the trip**

Keep a food journal or capture moments with photos. By documenting your culinary journey during pregnancy, you can later return to these memories and share them with your baby, creating a unique story about the nutrition he received even before birth.

7. **Traditions and rituals**

Create food-related traditions and rituals. Whether it's a weekly family dinner or a special dish you prepare for special occasions, these practices help create lasting memories of the joy of anticipation and togetherness.

8. **Educate and Engage**
Educate yourself about nutritional needs during pregnancy and involve your loved ones in the process. Sharing this knowledge will not only empower you but also create a supportive environment that values the importance of healthy, real food.

By increasing your intentional approach to food during pregnancy, you not only nourish your body but also set the stage for lifelong positive associations with healthy, real food for you and your baby.

RECIPES FOR FAMILY AND MATERNITY MILESTONES

Embarking on the journey of parenthood is a major milestone, and what better way to celebrate than with the joy of food? Whether you're expecting a new addition to your family or celebrating special moments with loved ones, these recipes are designed to add some culinary joy to your family and motherhood milestones.

1. **Pregnancy Announcement Pancakes**
 - Start the party with a sweet surprise by making heart-shaped crests and revealing your exciting news over breakfast. Add a dollop of whipped cream and some berries to add to the fun.

2. **Gender Cookies**
 - Create a set of cookies with a hidden color inside to reveal the gender of your baby. Watch as your family and friends discover a delightful secret with every bite.

3. **Baby Shower Brunch Quiche**
 - Throw an adorable baby shower brunch that includes a selection of mini pies. Offer a variety

of toppings, such as spinach and feta or bacon and cheddar, to satisfy all taste buds.

4. **Mocktails for expectant mothers**
 - A selection of refreshing cocktails for the mother expecting a toast. Create a "Mother Mojito" with mint, lime, and mineral water or a "Berry Bliss" with berries and ginger beer.

5. **Dad's signature dish**
 - Encourage the father-to-be to show off his culinary skills by preparing his dish for the family. It can become a cherished tradition as you celebrate milestones together.

6. **First family dinner**
 - Remember the first dinner as a family with a comforting and rich meal. Consider making a slow-cooked casserole or vegetable lasagna, and taking it all to dinner.

7. **Baby's first solid meal**
 - Capture the moment your baby eats his first piece of solid food. Puree fruits or vegetables and share this delightful experience with family members who will witness this sweet milestone.

8. **Monthly Milestone Cake**

- Celebrate your child and the first year of each month with a small cake specially designed for him. Let them dig in and create a fun and messy photo to cherish for years.

9. Grandpa's secret recipe
 - Get the grandparents involved by asking them to share a beloved family recipe. Prepare this special dish together, creating a bond between generations and building family traditions.

10. Family Recipe Diary
 - Document these culinary celebrations by creating a family recipe journal. Add used pictures, anecdotes, and recipes for each milestone and create a treasured memory for generations to come.

These recipes will not only nourish the body but also the soul, making your family and motherhood even more memorable. From the happy announcement to the first family dinner, enjoy every moment with delicious dishes that bring everyone together in the festive spirit.

CHAPTER 10
NUTRITIONAL GUIDELINES

Nutritional guidelines for real food during pregnancy are essential to ensure the health and well-being of both the mother and the developing baby. Here are some key recommendations for incorporating nutrient-dense, real foods into a pregnancy diet:

1. Fruits and Vegetables
   - Prioritize a colorful array of fruits and vegetables to provide a variety of vitamins, minerals, and antioxidants. Aim for at least five servings per day.

2. Whole Grains
   - Choose whole grains like brown rice, quinoa, oats, and whole wheat bread for a rich source of fiber, B vitamins, and sustained energy.

3. Lean Proteins
   - Include lean protein sources such as poultry, lean meats, fish, eggs, and plant-based options like beans and lentils. Protein is crucial for the baby's growth and development.

4. Dairy or Dairy Alternatives

- Opt for low-fat or fat-free dairy products or fortified plant-based alternatives to ensure an adequate intake of calcium for bone development.

5. Healthy Fats

- Incorporate sources of healthy fats like avocados, nuts, seeds, and olive oil. Omega-3 fatty acids, found in fatty fish, are particularly important for the baby's brain and eye development.

6. Iron-Rich Foods

- Include iron-rich foods such as lean meats, poultry, fish, beans, and lentils to prevent iron deficiency and support the increased blood volume during pregnancy.

7. Folate/Folic Acid Sources

- Ensure sufficient intake of folate from sources like leafy greens, citrus fruits, and fortified grains to reduce the risk of neural tube defects.

8. Hydration

- Stay well-hydrated by drinking plenty of water throughout the day. Proper hydration is essential for supporting increased blood volume and preventing dehydration.

9. **Limit Processed and Sugary Foods**

- Minimize the consumption of processed foods, sugary snacks, and beverages. Instead, focus on nutrient-dense options to meet the increased nutritional demands.

10. **Moderate Caffeine and Avoid Alcohol**

- Limit caffeine intake and completely avoid alcohol during pregnancy, as they can have potential adverse effects on the developing baby.

11. **Small, Frequent Meals**

- Opt for smaller, more frequent meals to manage nausea and maintain steady blood sugar levels.

12. **Listen to Your Body**

- Pay attention to hunger and fullness cues. Eat when hungry, and stop when satisfied.

Remember, these guidelines are general recommendations, and it's crucial to consult with healthcare professionals for personalized advice based on individual health conditions and needs. Every pregnancy is unique, and a healthcare provider can provide tailored guidance to ensure a healthy and well-balanced diet throughout this special time.

KITCHEN FOR REAL FOOD PREGNANCY

Creating a truly edible pregnancy kitchen requires prioritizing nutrient-dense whole foods to support the health and well-being of both mother and child. Here are some key considerations.

1. Emphasis on whole foods
 - Choose healthy, unprocessed foods such as fruits, vegetables, whole grains, lean proteins and healthy fats.

- Choose organic options when possible to reduce exposure to pesticides.

2. Rich Nutrients
 - Add a variety of colorful fruits and vegetables to ensure a wide range of vitamins and minerals.

- Include sources of iron, calcium, folic acid, and omega-3 fatty acids, which are important for fetal development.

3. Balanced meals
 - Aim for a balanced meal that includes a mix of carbohydrates, proteins, and fats.

- Choose complex carbohydrates such as whole grains to provide sustained energy.

4. **Hydration is the key**
 - Stay well hydrated with water, herbal tea, and natural fruit juices.

- Limit caffeine and avoid alcohol during pregnancy.

5. **Food preparation and planning**
 - Plan and prepare meals to ensure a constant supply of nutrients.

- Consider baking and freezing portions for convenient and healthy options.

6. **Smart snack**
 - Choose nutritious snacks such as nuts, seeds, yogurt, and fresh fruit.

- Avoid overly processed snacks that are high in added sugar and unhealthy fats.

7. **Protein intake**
 - Include lean protein sources in your meals, such as poultry, fish, beans, and tofu.

- Adequate protein content supports fetal tissue growth.

8. **Supplements**
 - Work with your doctor to determine what prenatal supplements you need, such as folic acid and iron.

9. **Mindful eating**
 - Practice mindful eating to enjoy and appreciate every bite.

- Pay attention to signs of hunger and satiety to avoid overeating.

10. **Food Safety**
 - Implement appropriate food safety measures to prevent foodborne illnesses.

- Avoid raw or undercooked meat and seafood.
   Remember that by consulting a doctor or nutritionist, you will receive personalized guidance during pregnancy based on individual health needs. It's important to have a well-stocked kitchen with the right tools and ingredients. Here are some essential supplies you will need:

- High-quality blender or food processor for making smoothies, sauces and more.

- A cast iron pan for cooking without toxic chemicals.

- Organic, grass-fed meat, wild-caught fish, and pastured eggs for optimal nutrition.

- Various vegetables, fruits, and herbs that add flavor and nutrition to food.

- High quality oils

- A good cutting board for chopping vegetables and other ingredients.

- Sharp knives for easy cutting and slicing.

- High-quality baking sheet for frying vegetables and baking healthy sweets.

   With the right tools and ingredients, you can prepare delicious and nutritious meals during pregnancy.

CHAPTER 11
DIRECTORY

1. Grocery Stores

- *Organic Market*
Check out your local organic market with a wide variety of fresh produce and make sure your pregnancy diet is rich in vitamins and minerals.

- *Specialty Health Shops*
Visit shops that focus on the health of organic fruits, nuts, and seeds and promote a varied and nutritious diet.

2. Farmer's market

- Locally Sourced Produce
Connect with local farmers for direct access to fresh fruits and vegetables, supporting both your health and your community.

3. Online Resources

- *Organic Food Delivery Services*
Take advantage of online platforms that deliver organic and natural food to your

doorstep with convenience without compromising on quality.

4. Nutritional supplements

- *Pharmacy*
Find a variety of prenatal vitamins and minerals to support nutritional needs during pregnancy at reputable pharmacies.

5. Restaurants and cafes

- Farm-to-Table Restaurants
Choose eateries that prioritize fresh, local ingredients so you can maintain a healthy and nutritious diet while dining out.

6. Cooking Lessons

- *Prenatal Cooking Workshops*
Attend courses that focus on preparing meals according to your pregnancy and provide valuable information on how to prepare delicious and nutritious meals.

7. Recipe Blogs

- *Nutrient-dense Recipes*

Discover pregnancy nutrition blogs that offer creative and delicious recipes that contain essential nutrients for you and your baby.

8. **Community Support**

- *Size Support Groups*
Join local or online pregnancy communities to exchange knowledge on where to find the best real food options and share meal ideas with like-minded people.

9. **Training programs**

- *Nutrition Courses*
Enroll in prenatal nutrition courses to deepen your understanding of specific nutritional needs during pregnancy, enabling you to make informed food choices.

10. **Books and manuals**

- *Prenatal Nutrition Books*
Read authoritative books and guides on real pregnancy nutrition for in-depth information on specific nutrients and the importance of meal planning.

Remember to ask your doctor for personal advice on your nutritional needs during pregnancy. This directory is a guide to help you navigate this crucial time and find the best sources of real, nutritious food.